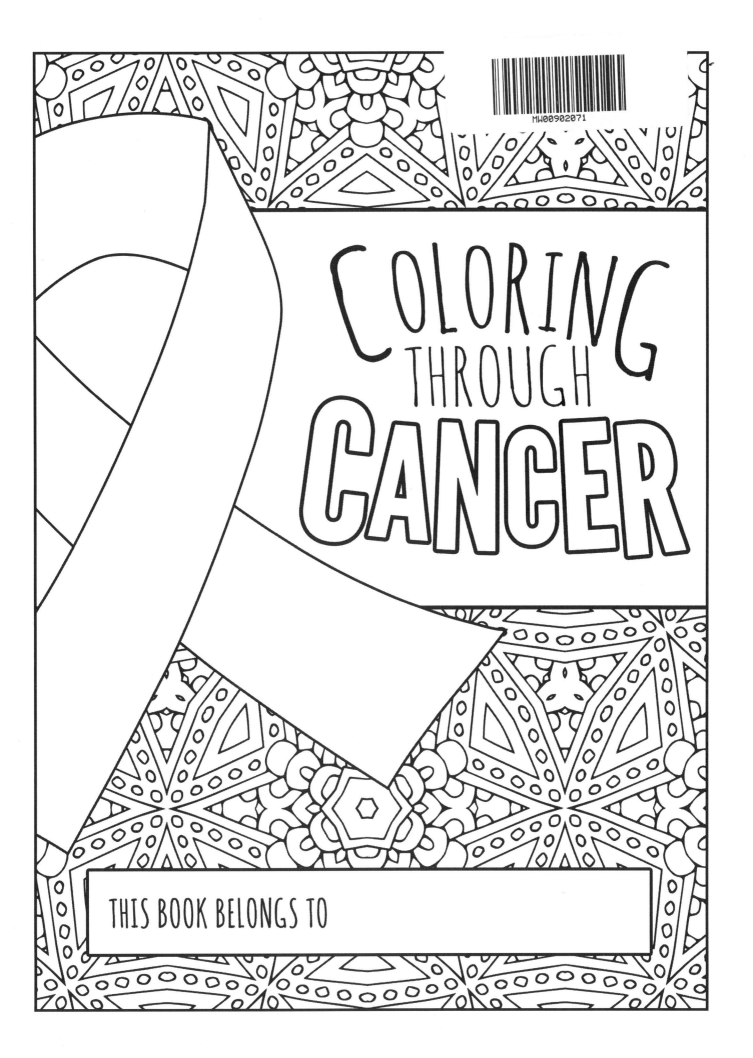

COLORING THROUGH CANCER

THIS BOOK BELONGS TO

I want to dedicate this book to my mom, Lyn.

Through the highs and lows of a life touched by cancer, you've
never stopped smiling and inspiring others.

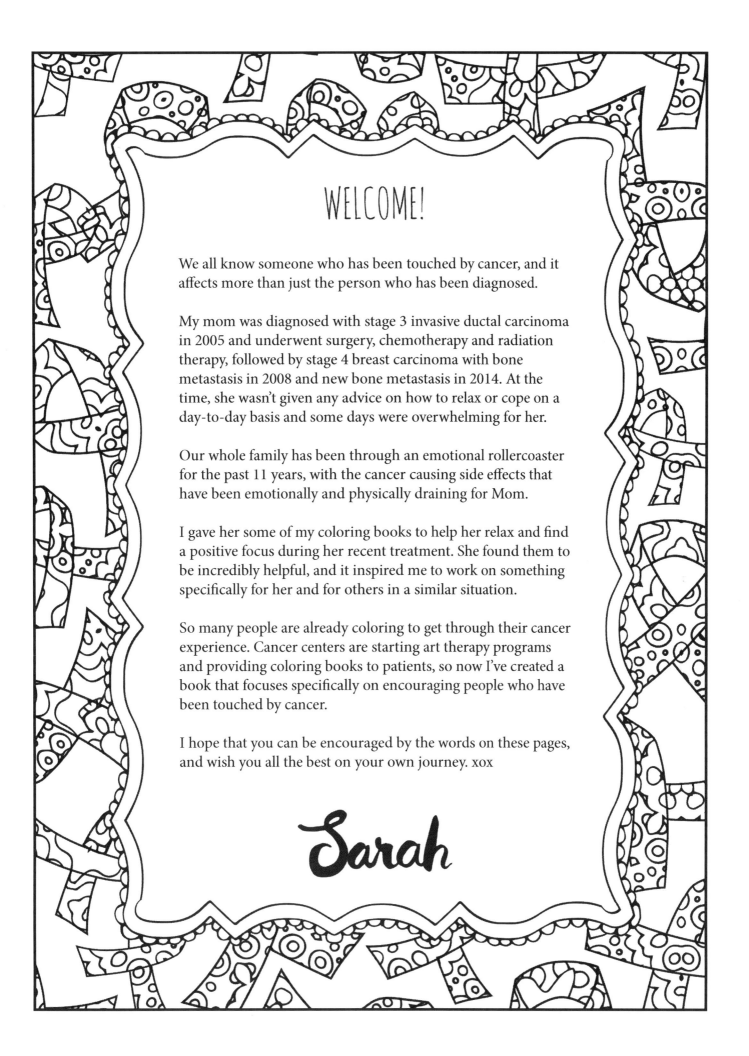

WELCOME!

We all know someone who has been touched by cancer, and it affects more than just the person who has been diagnosed.

My mom was diagnosed with stage 3 invasive ductal carcinoma in 2005 and underwent surgery, chemotherapy and radiation therapy, followed by stage 4 breast carcinoma with bone metastasis in 2008 and new bone metastasis in 2014. At the time, she wasn't given any advice on how to relax or cope on a day-to-day basis and some days were overwhelming for her.

Our whole family has been through an emotional rollercoaster for the past 11 years, with the cancer causing side effects that have been emotionally and physically draining for Mom.

I gave her some of my coloring books to help her relax and find a positive focus during her recent treatment. She found them to be incredibly helpful, and it inspired me to work on something specifically for her and for others in a similar situation.

So many people are already coloring to get through their cancer experience. Cancer centers are starting art therapy programs and providing coloring books to patients, so now I've created a book that focuses specifically on encouraging people who have been touched by cancer.

I hope that you can be encouraged by the words on these pages, and wish you all the best on your own journey. xox

Sarah

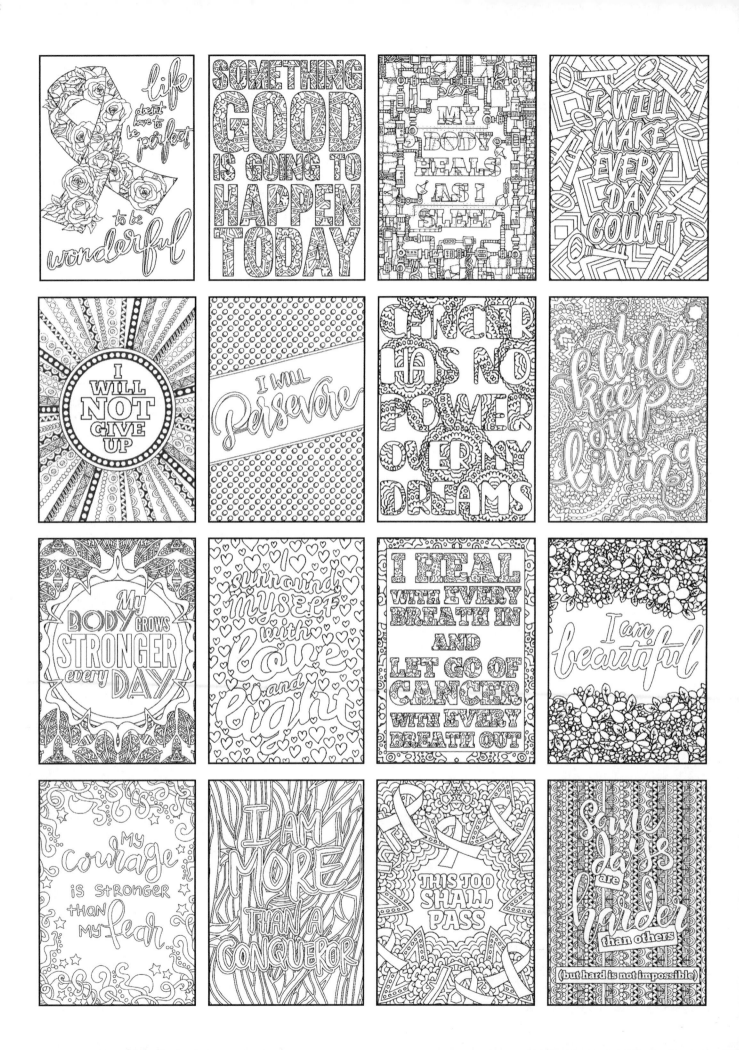

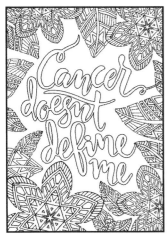

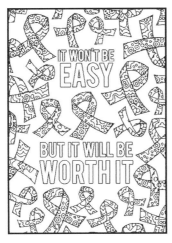

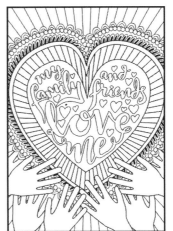

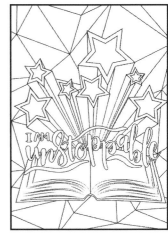

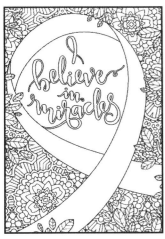

SHARE YOUR JOURNEY

Share your story and colored pages with others who are coloring through cancer
#coloringthroughcancer

Join our coloring community

facebook.com/groups/coloringthroughcancer

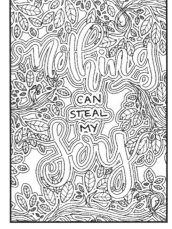

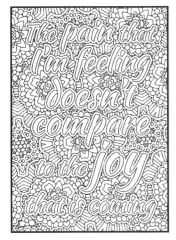

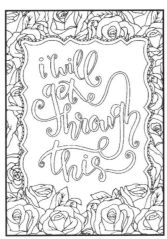

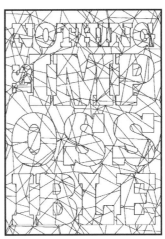

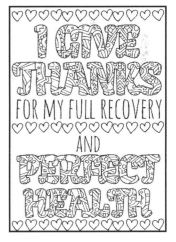

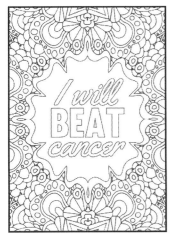

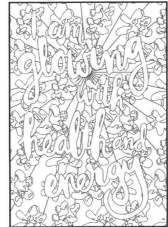

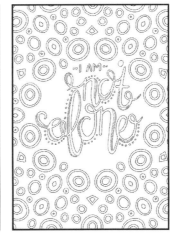

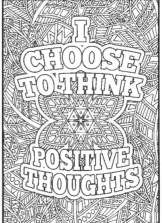

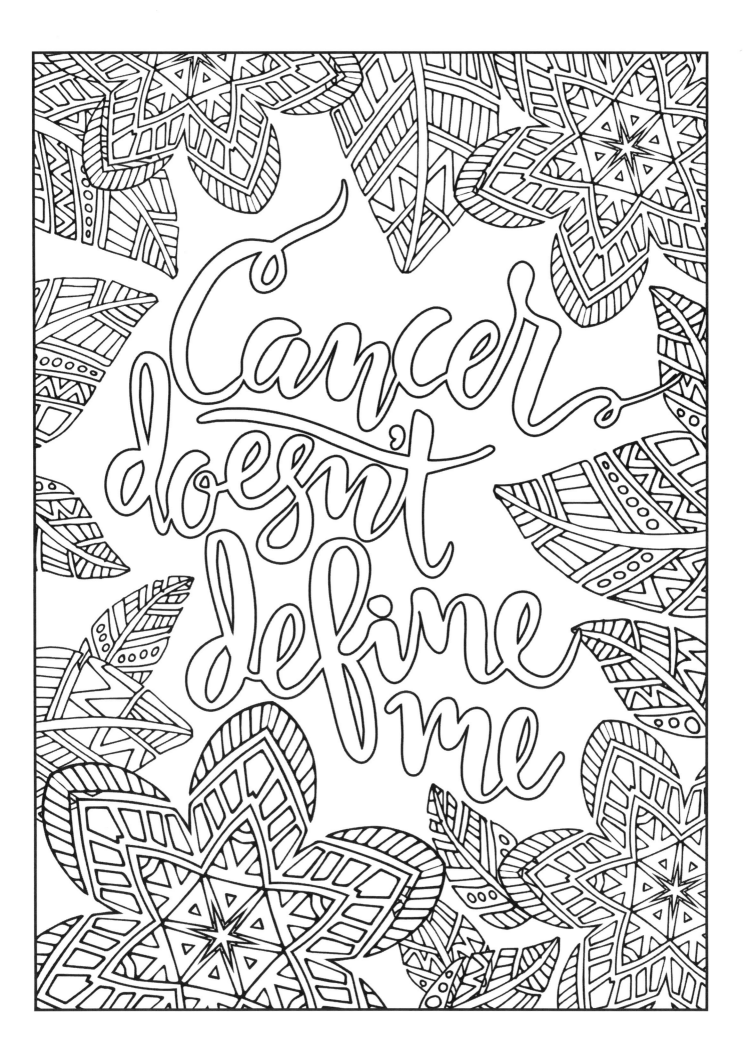

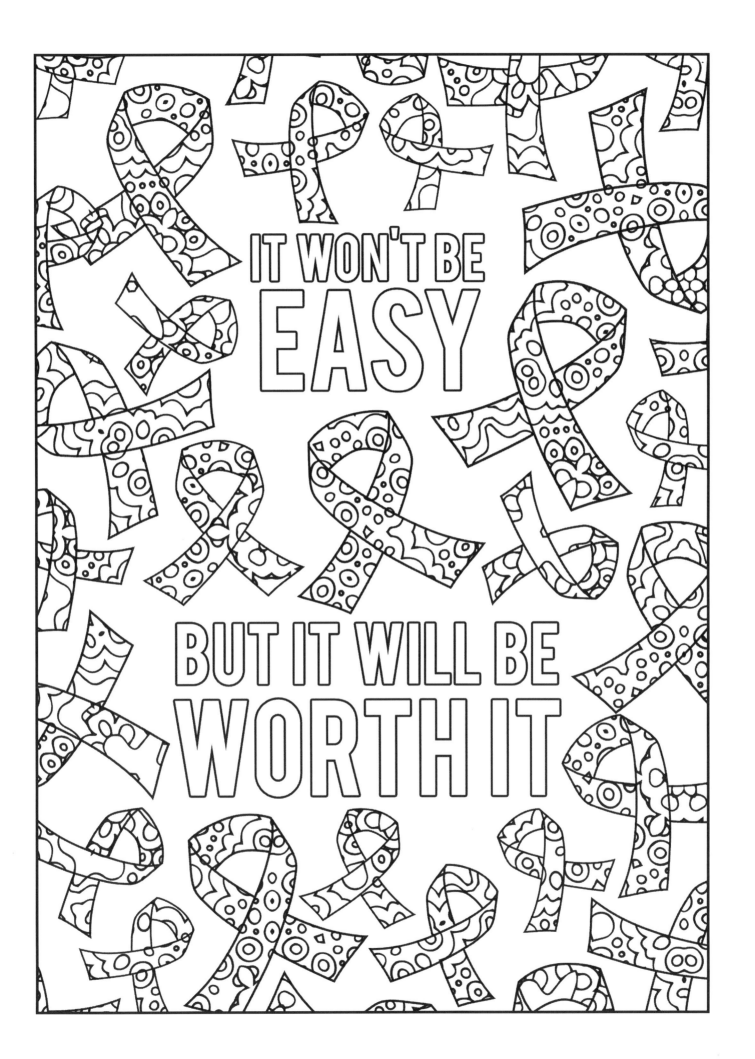

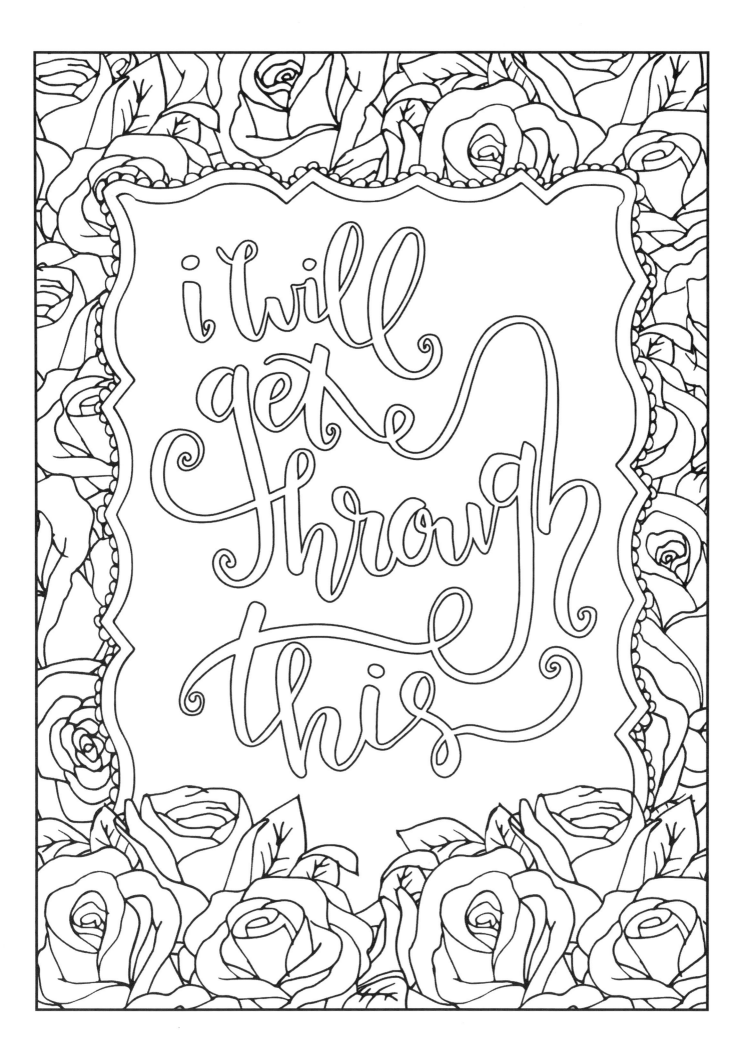

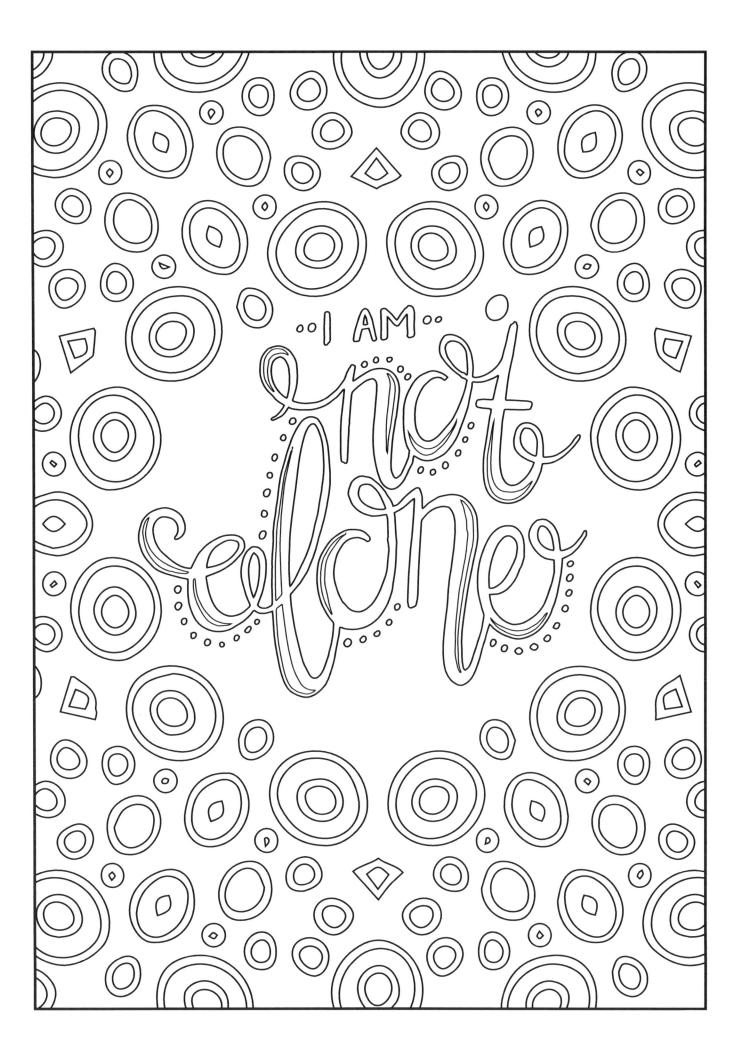

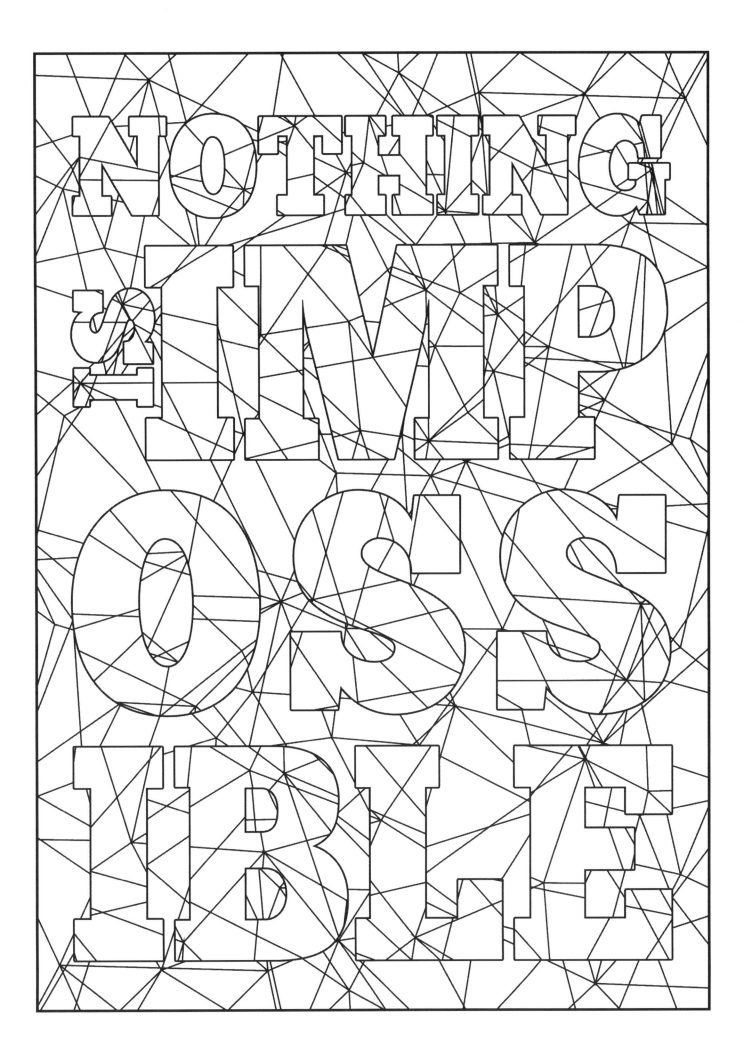

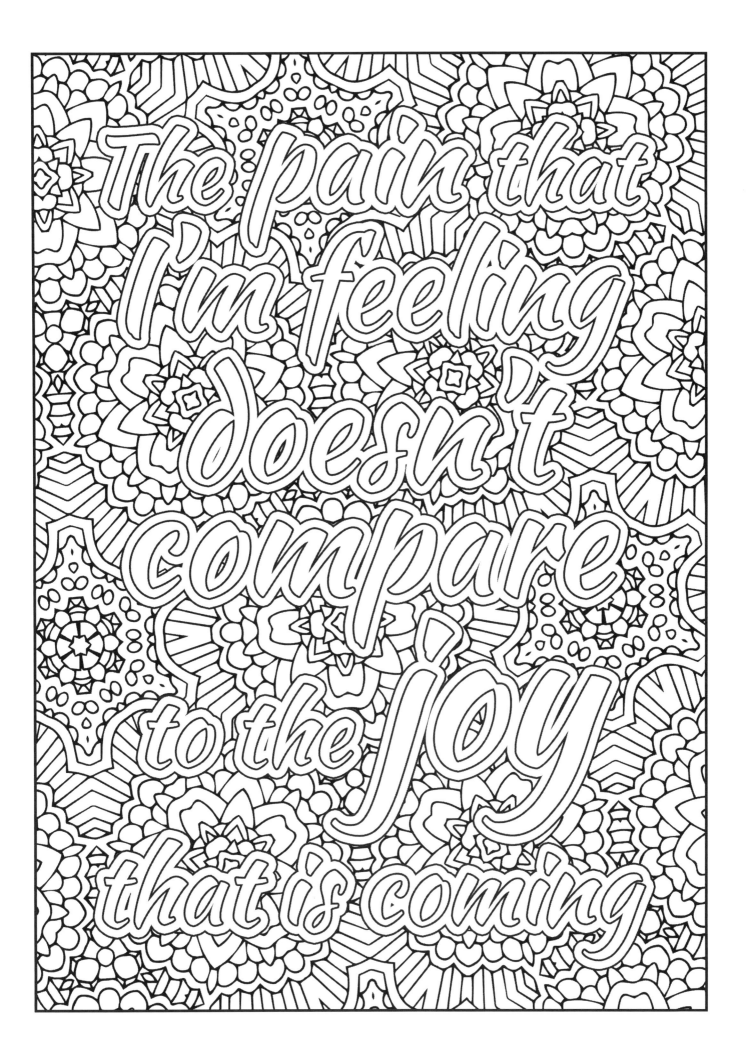

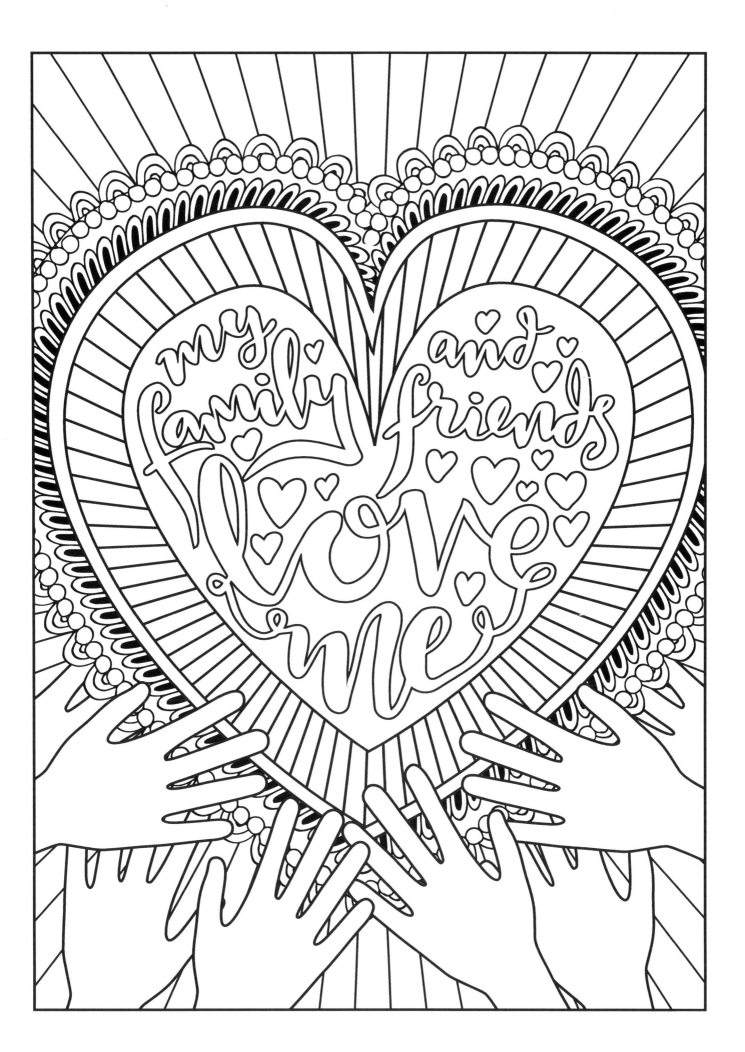

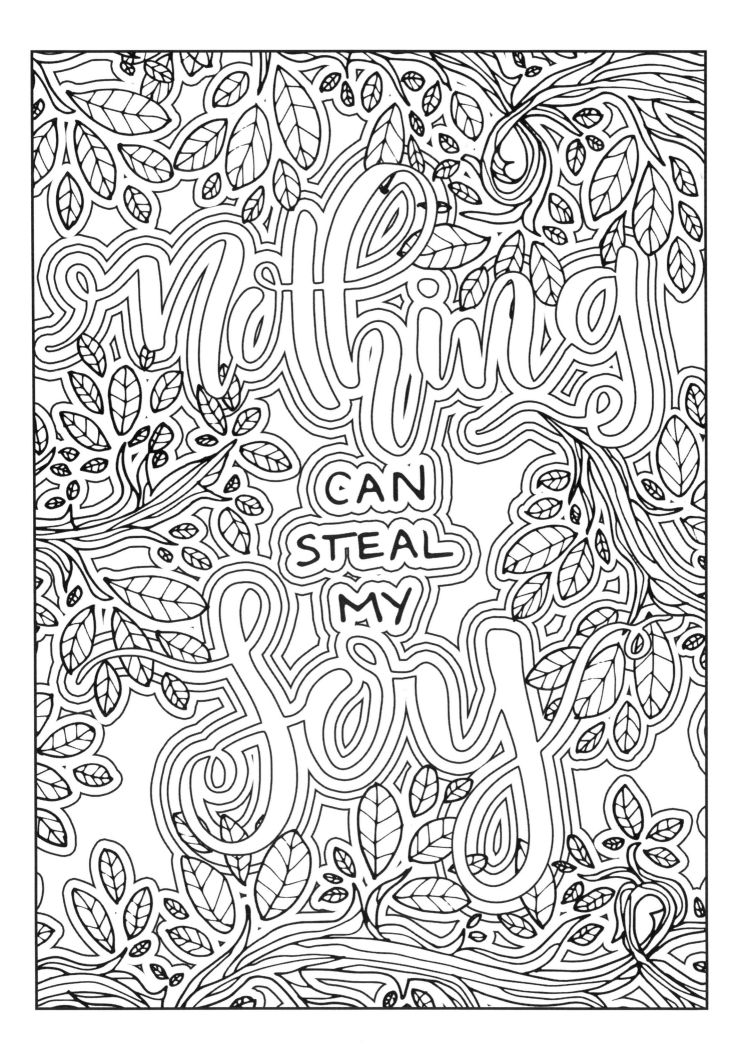

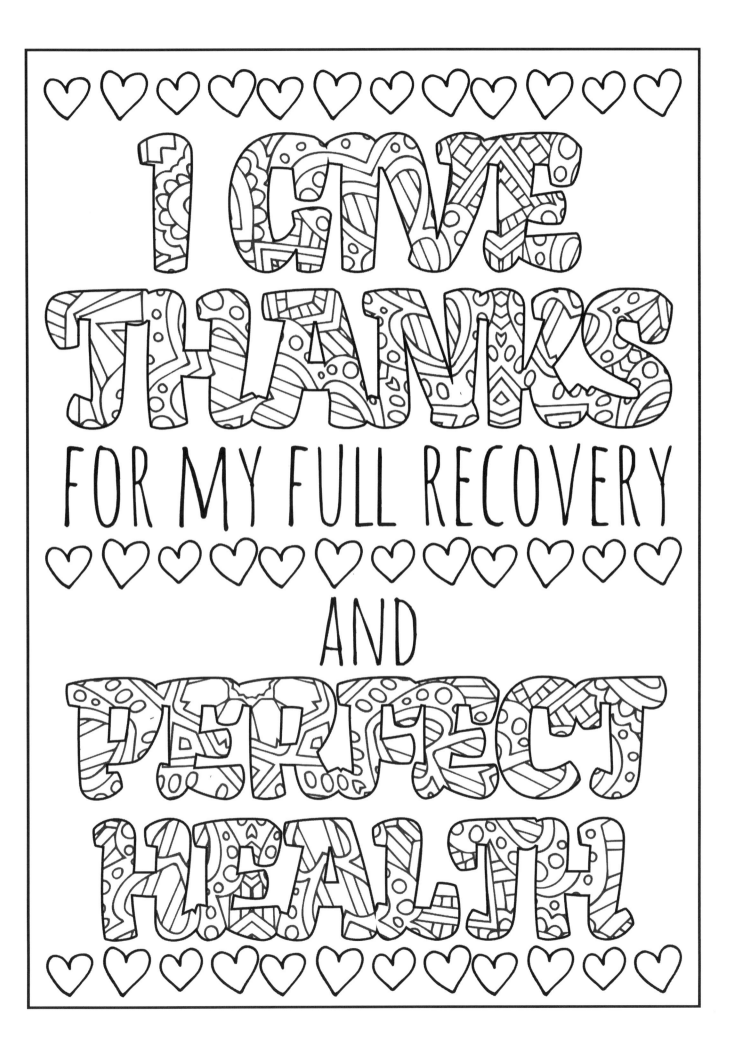

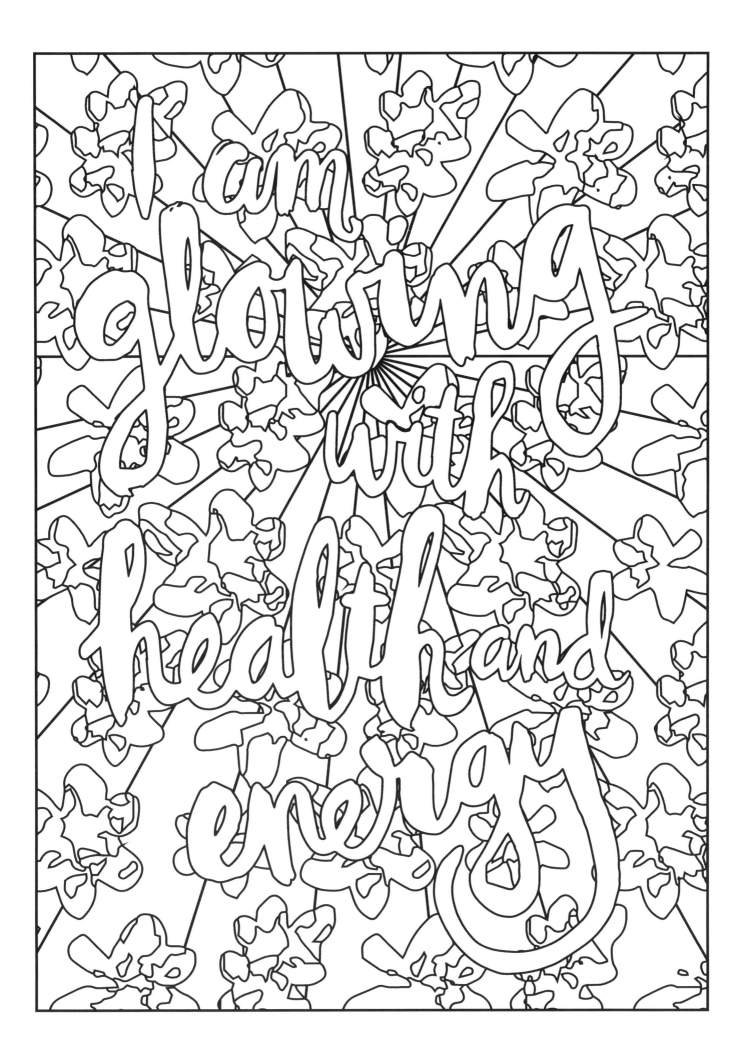

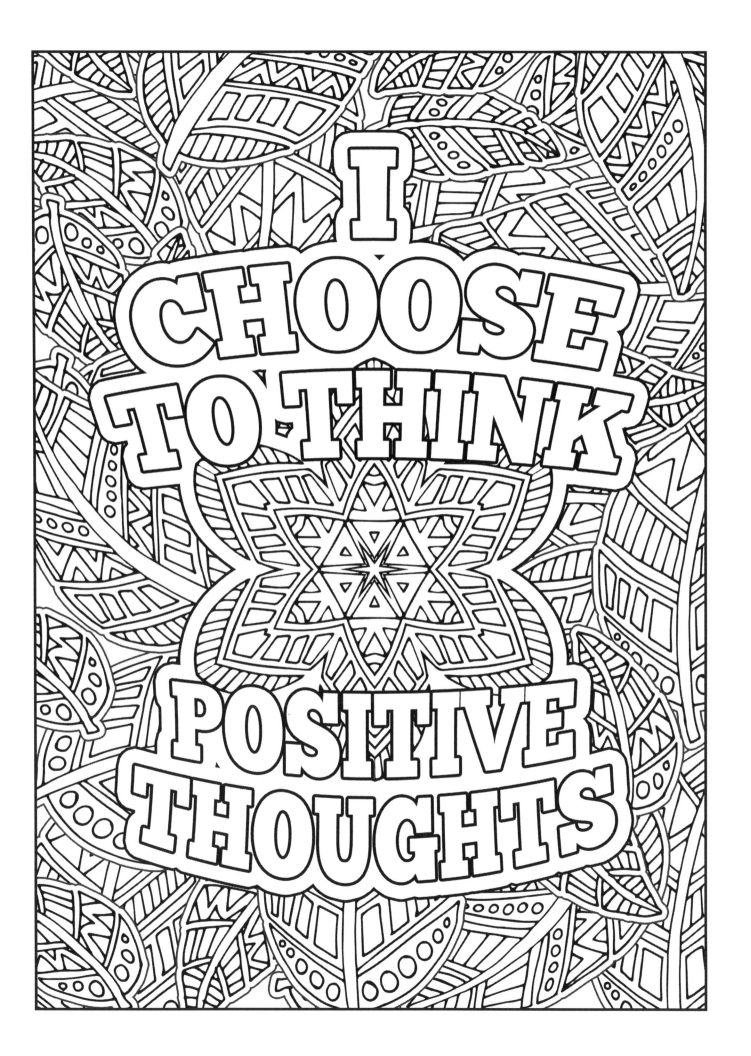

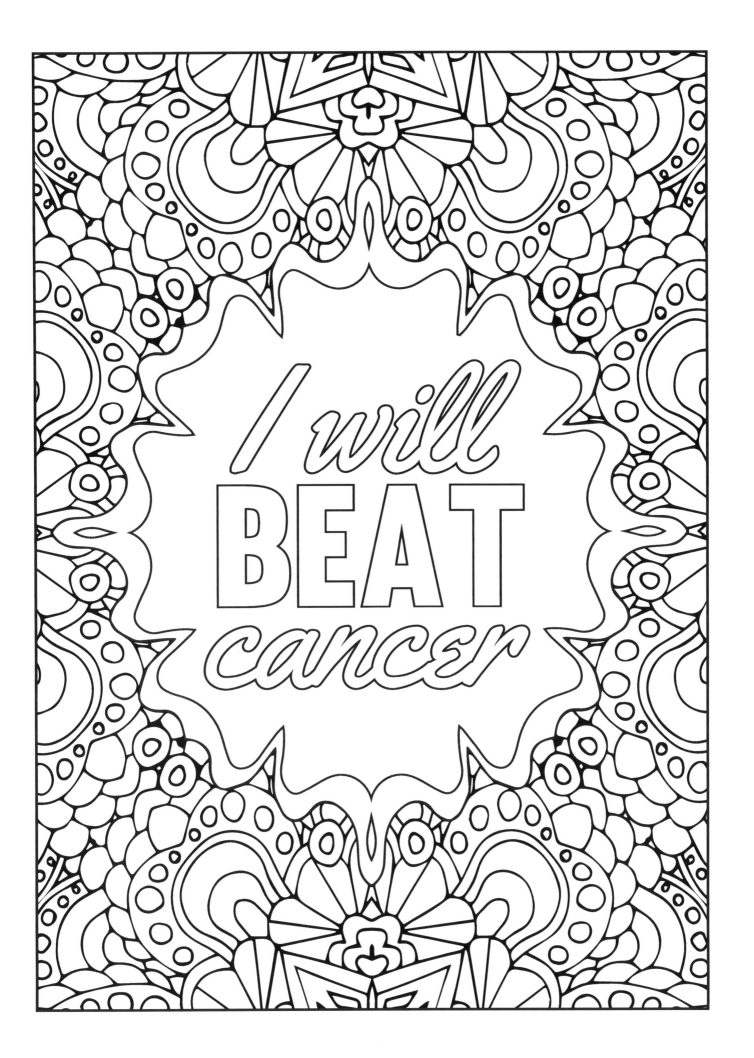

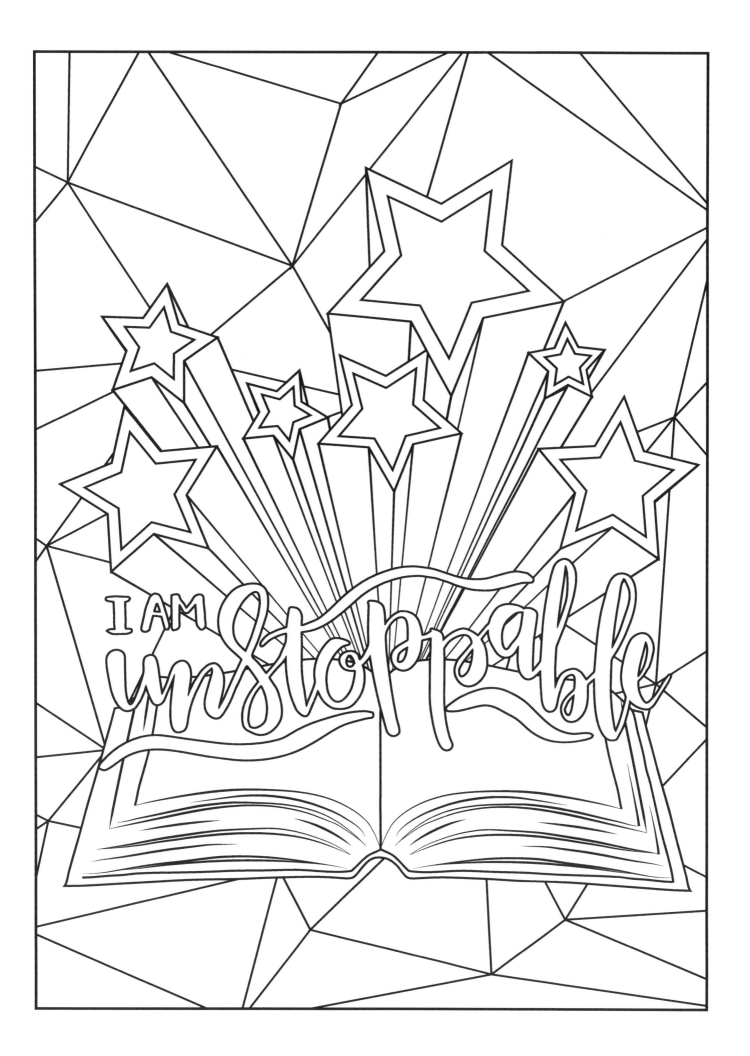

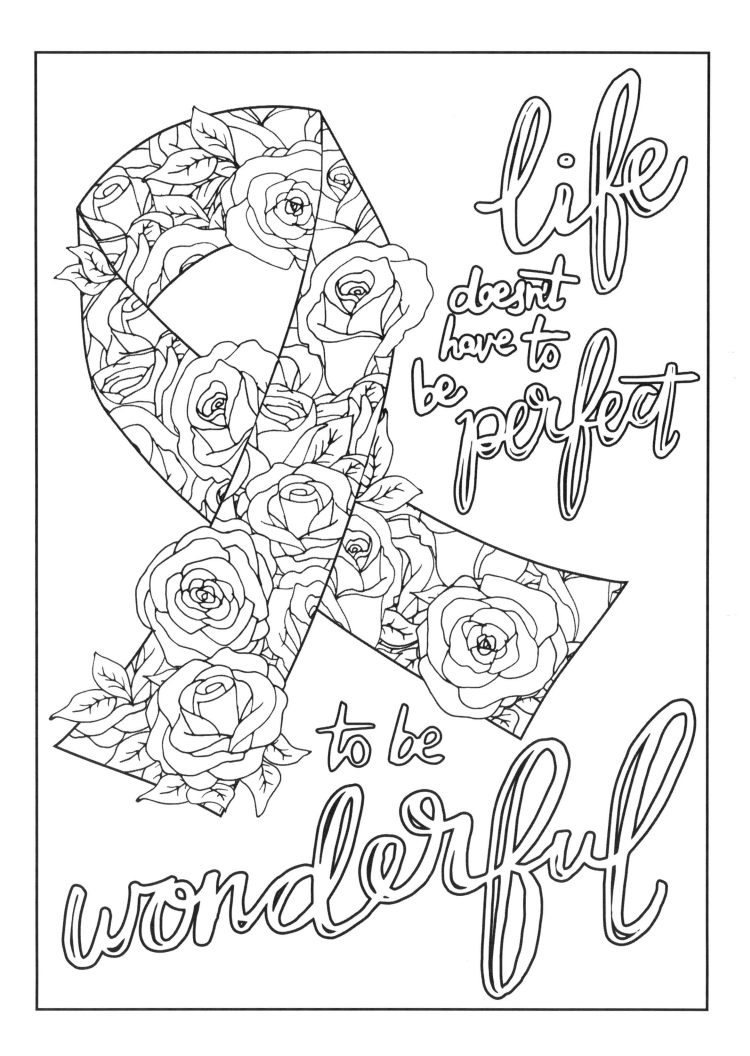

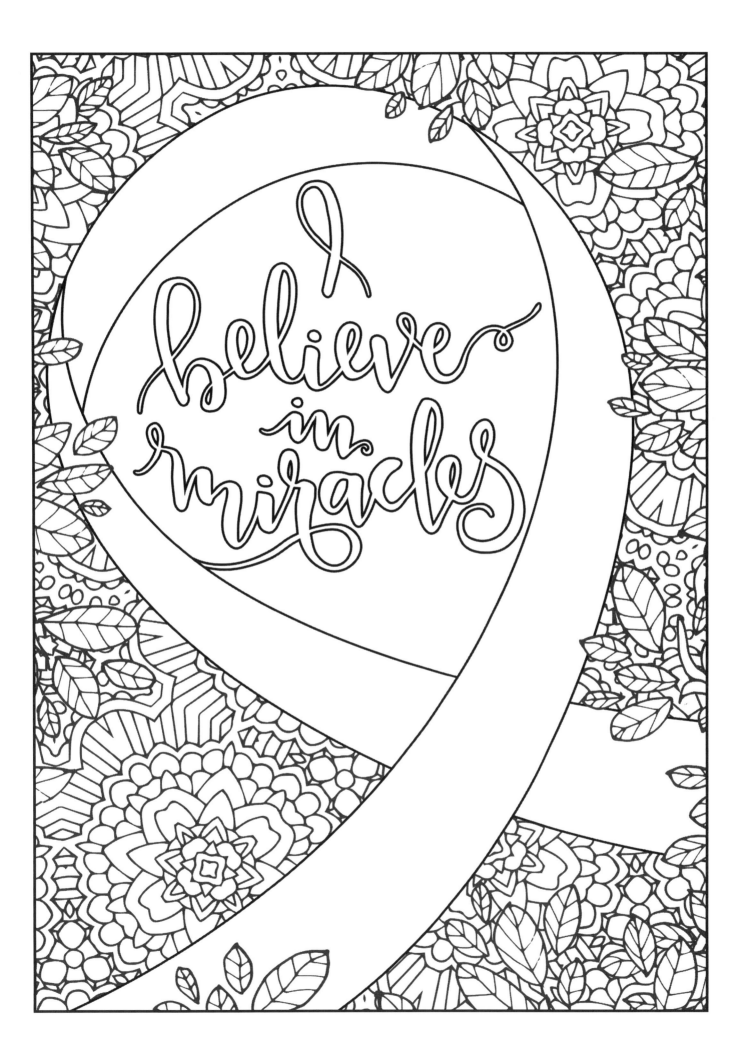

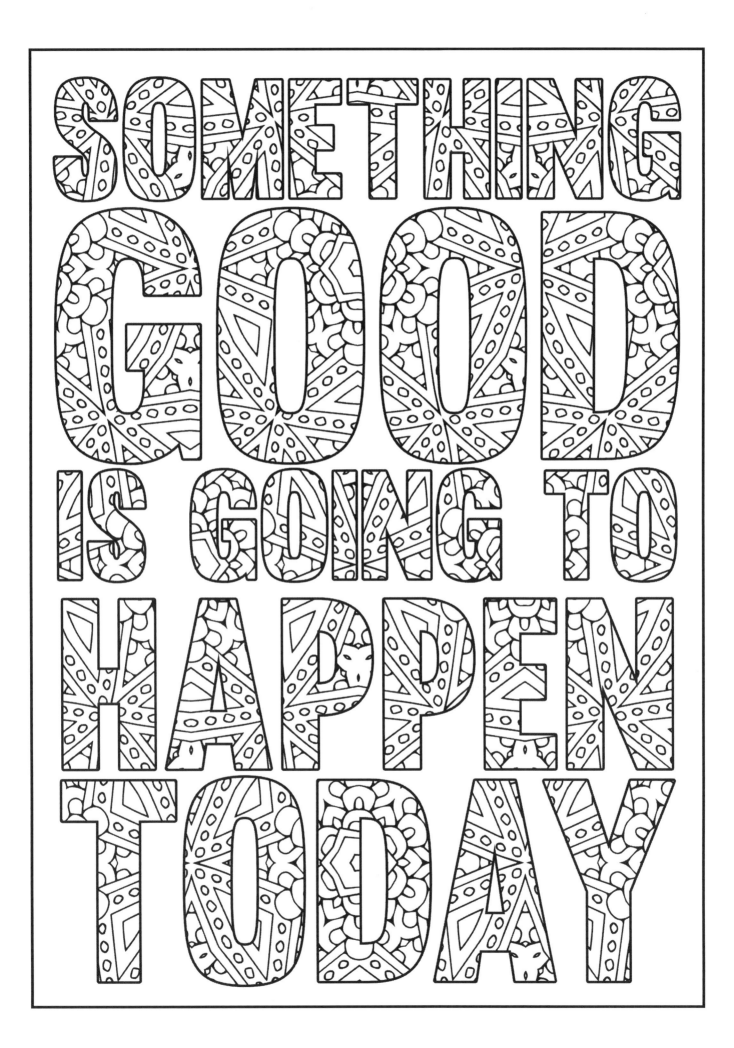

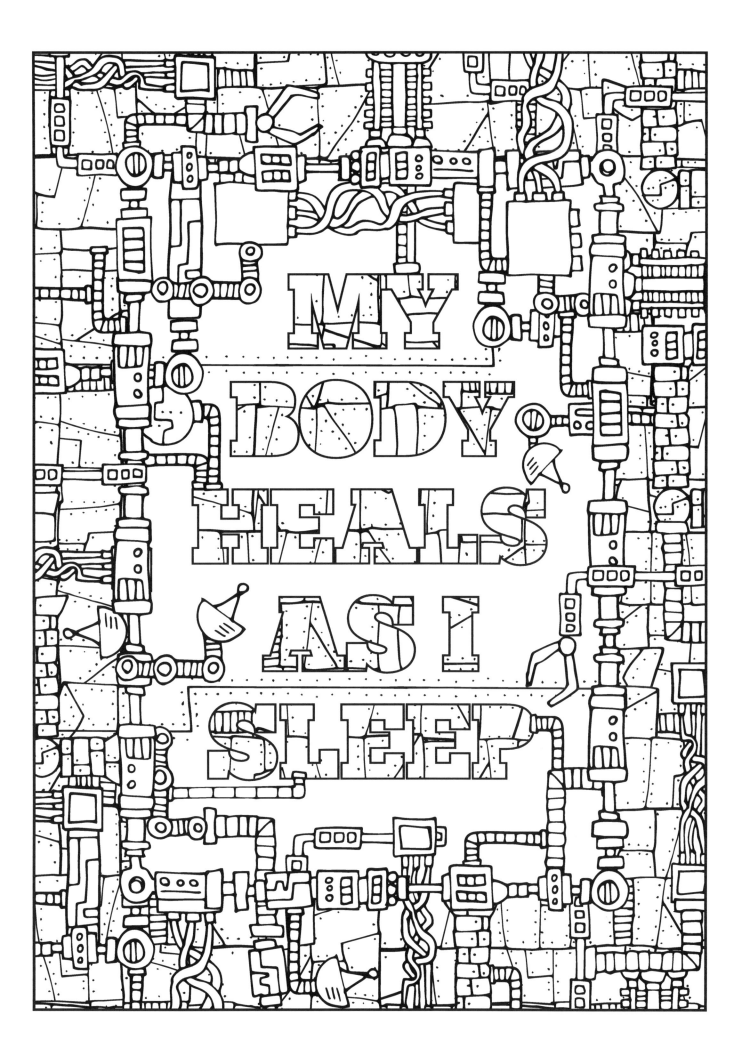

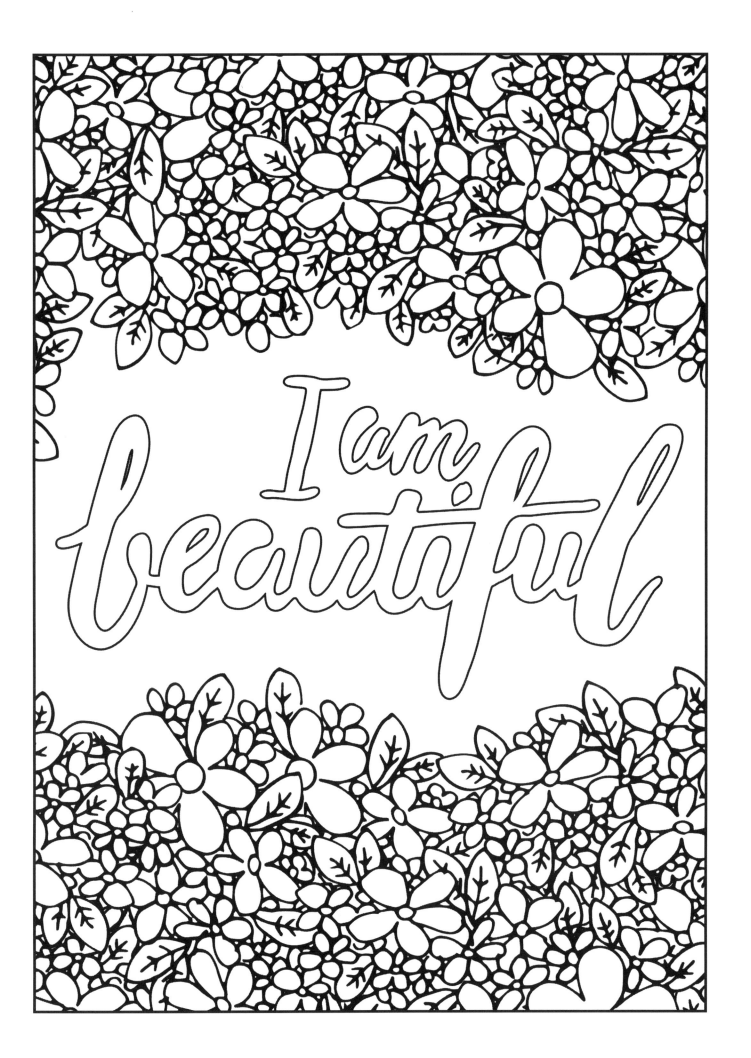

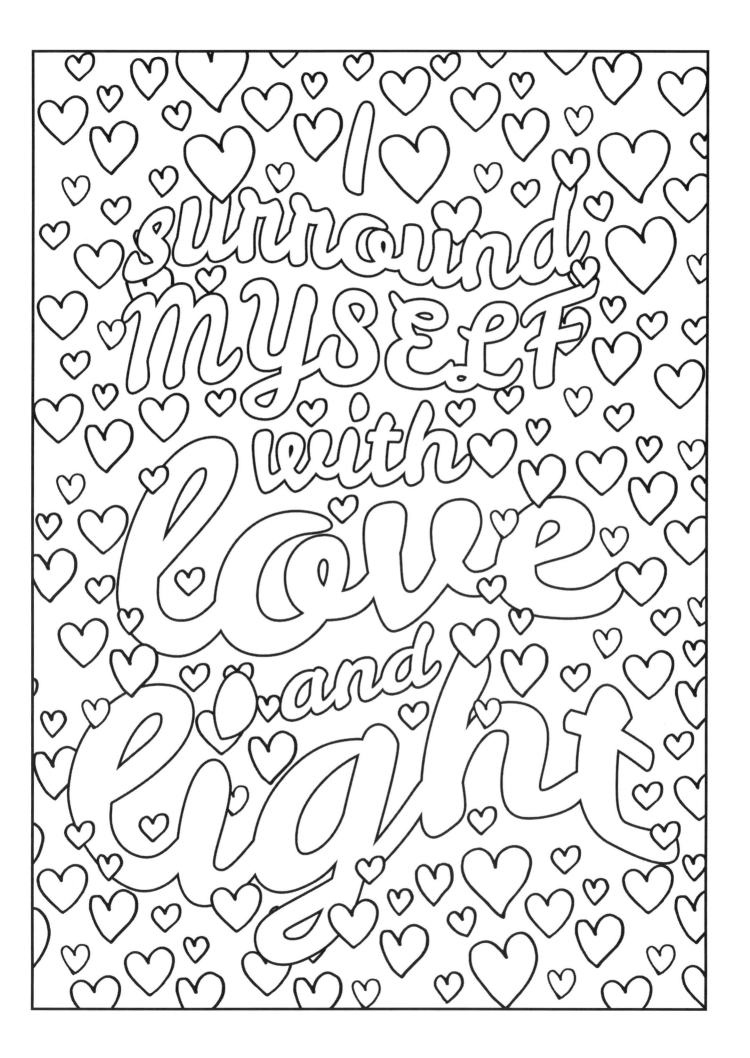

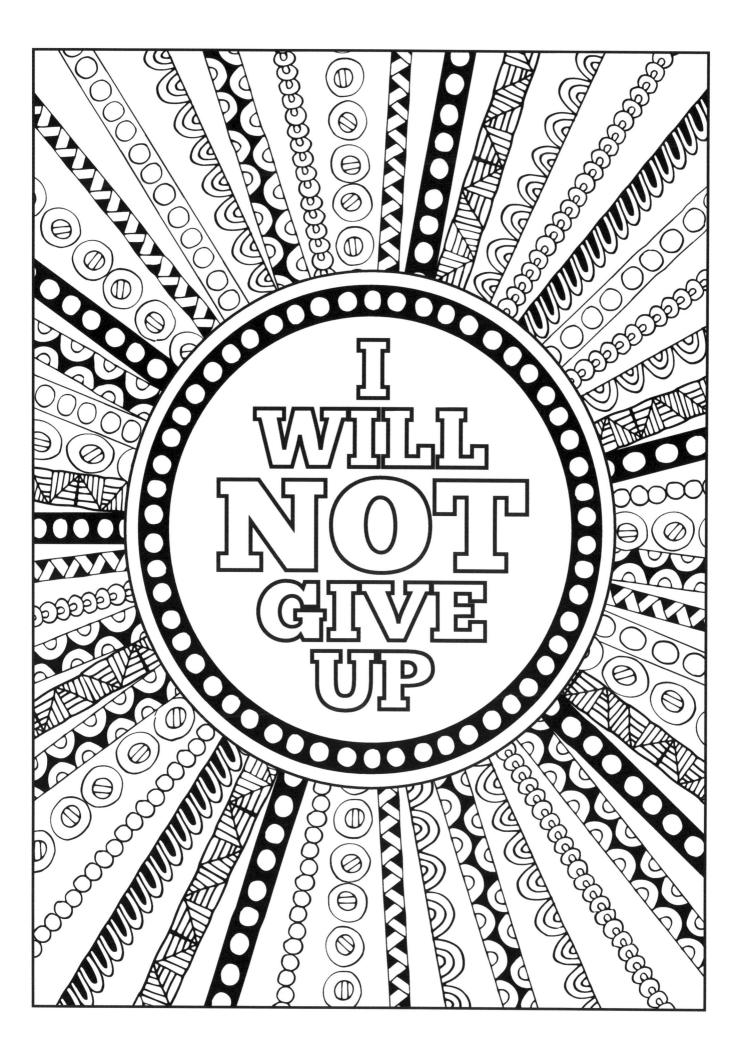

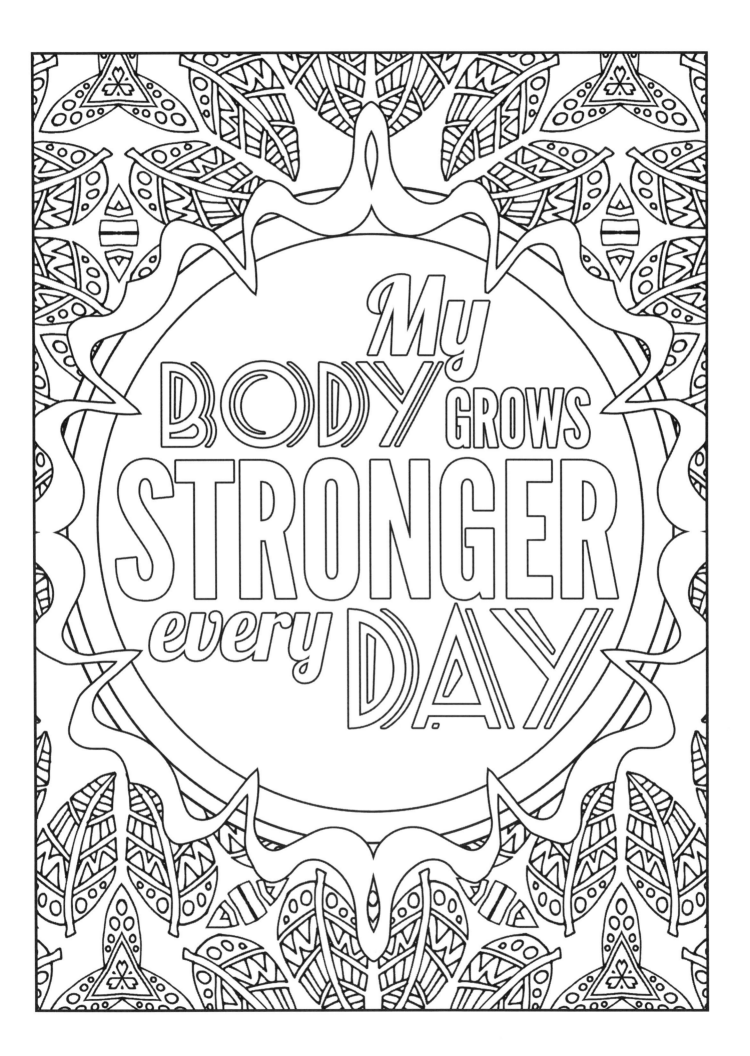

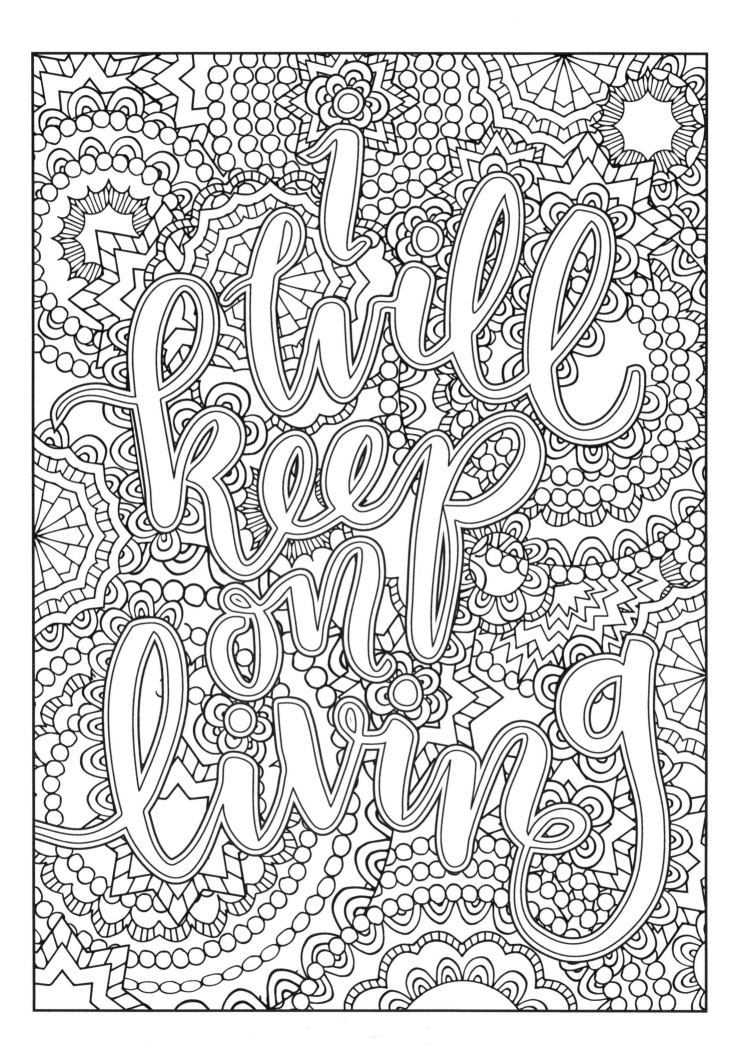

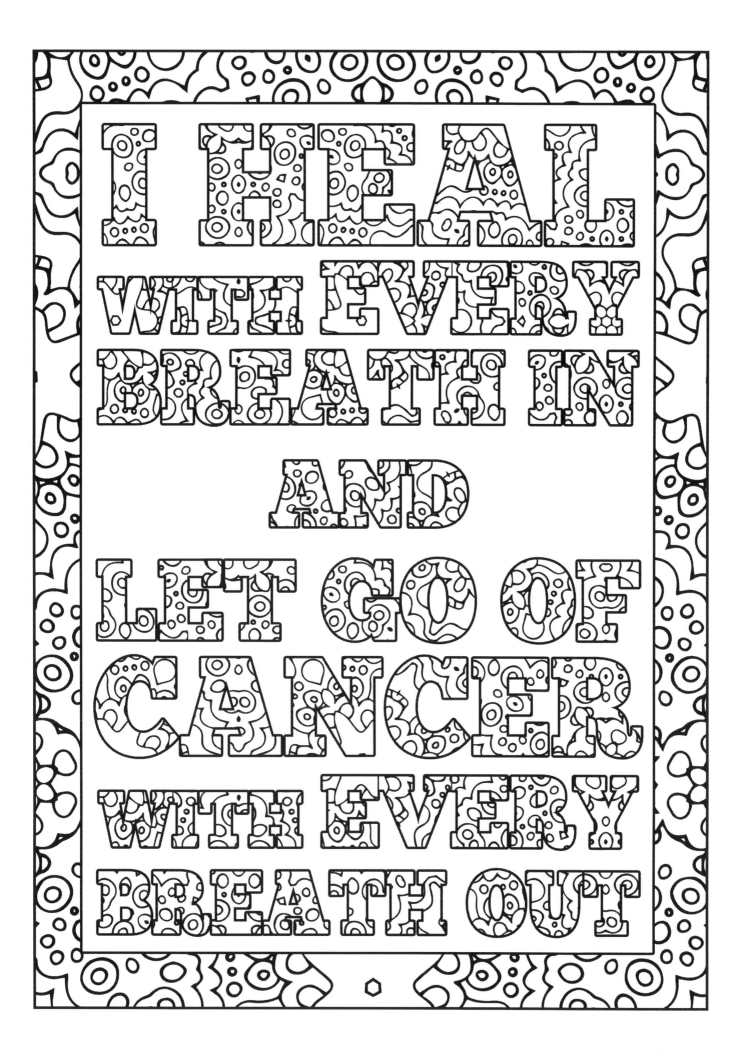

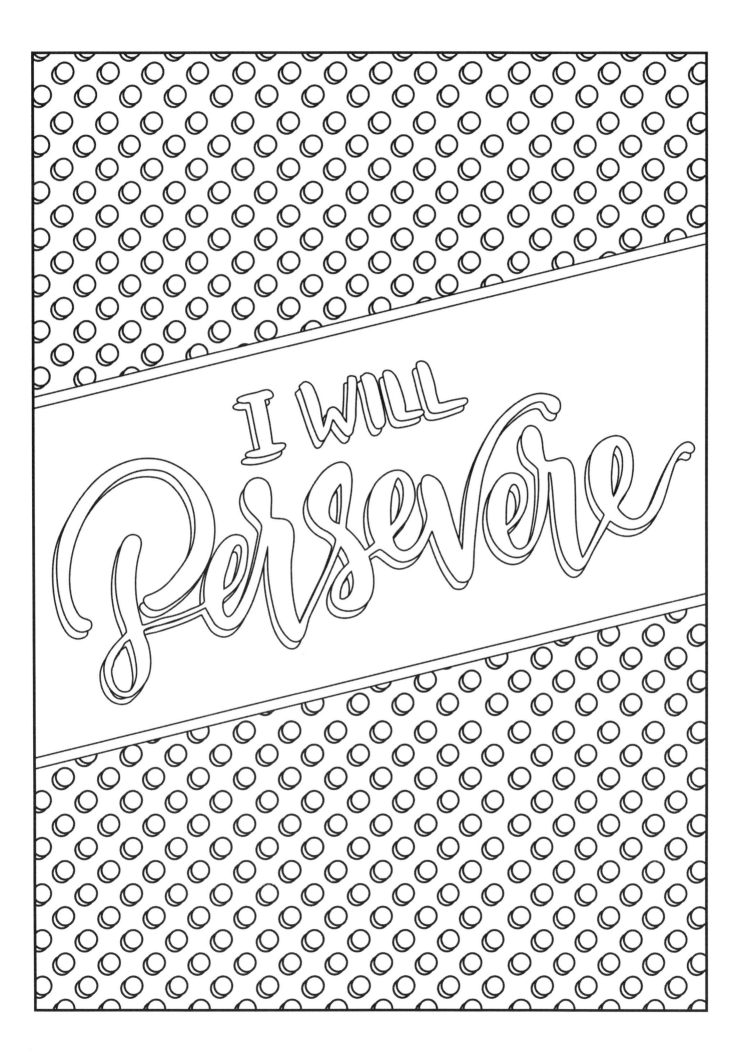

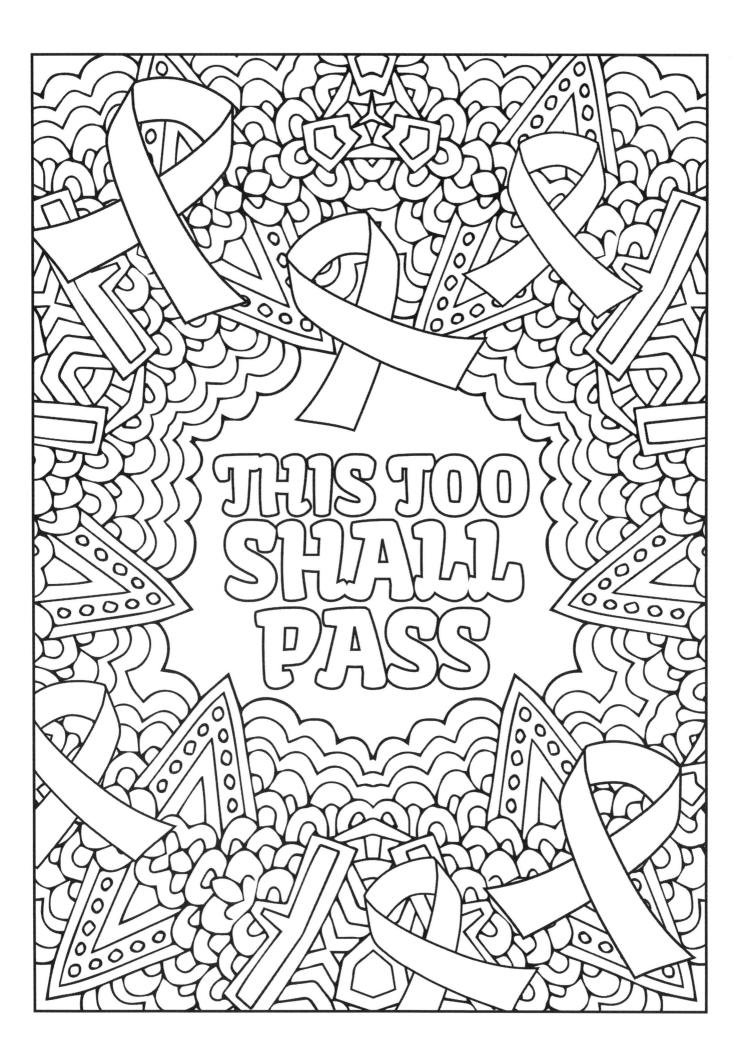

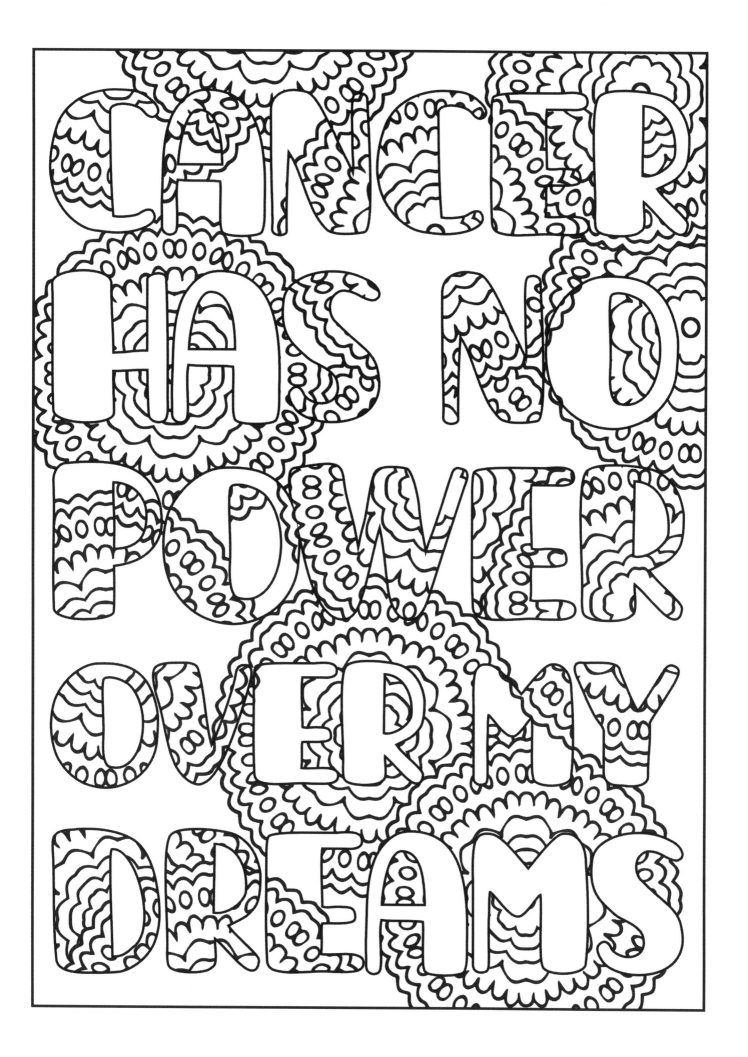

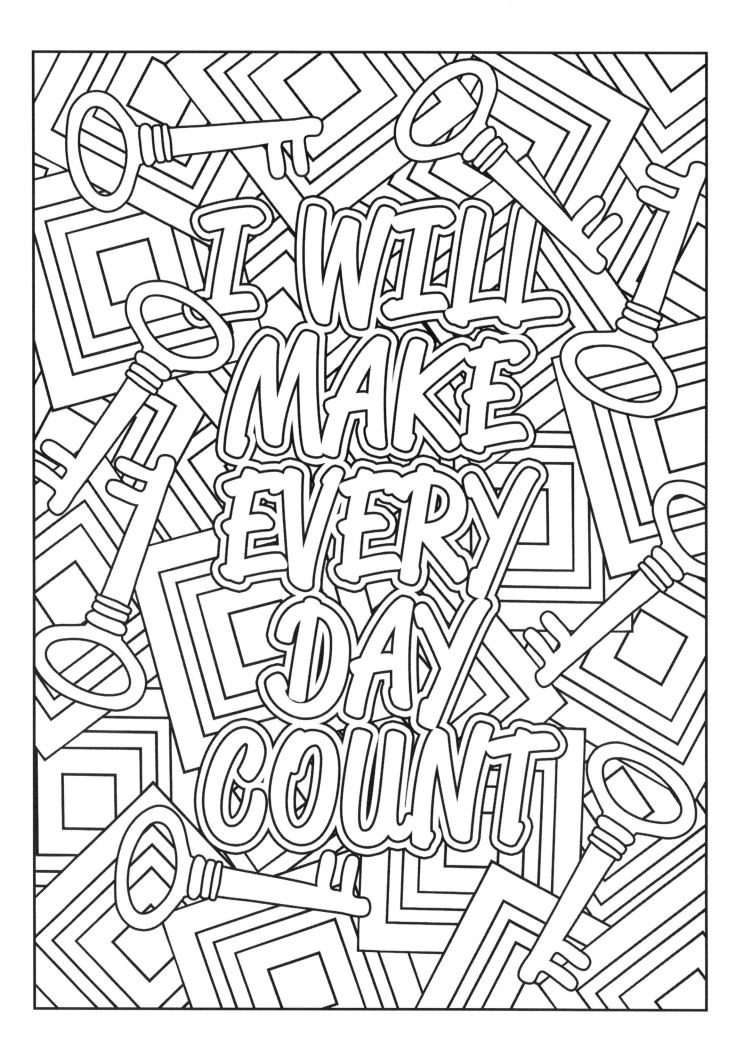

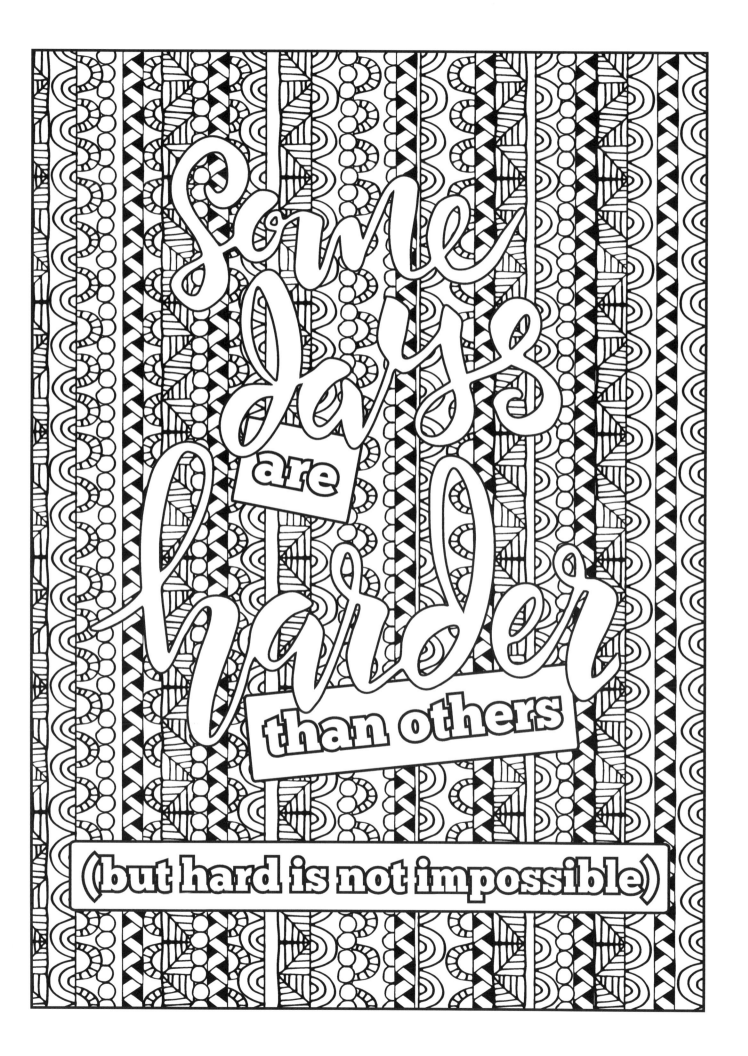

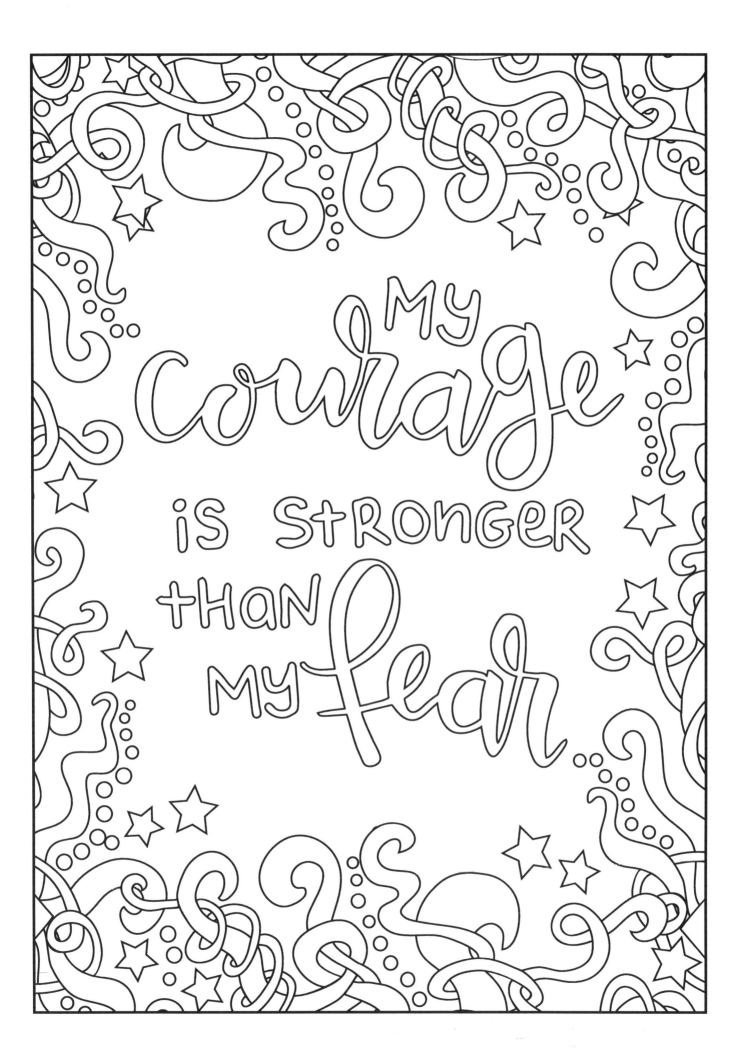

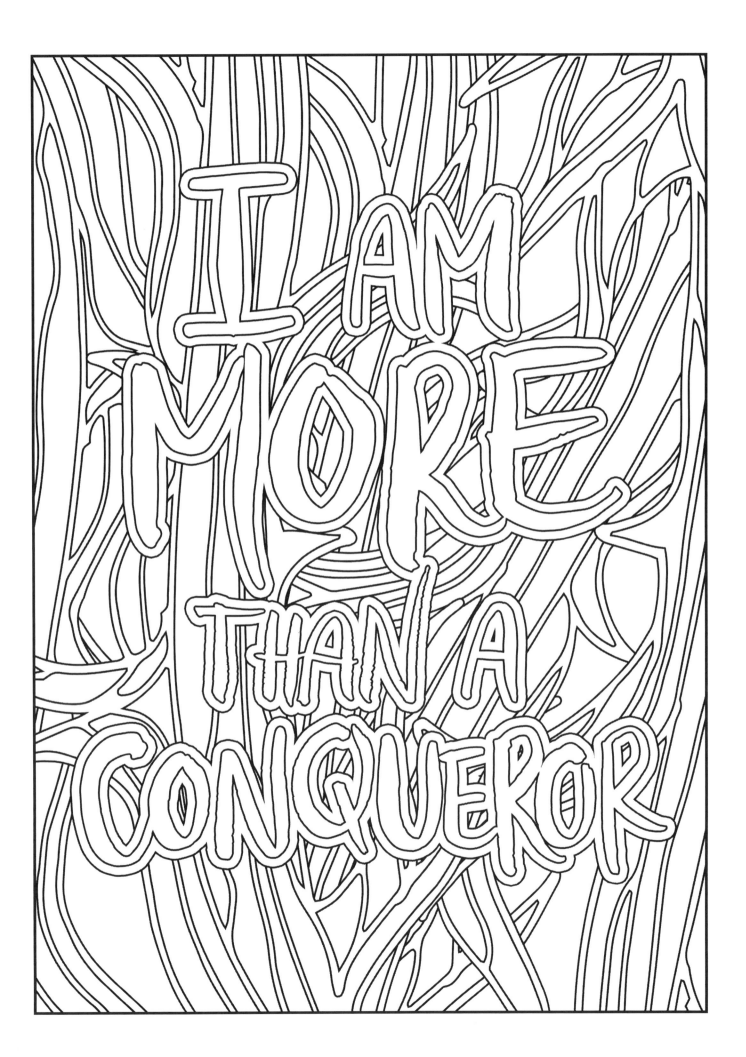

USE THIS COLOR WHEEL TO COMPARE COLORS AND SHADES!

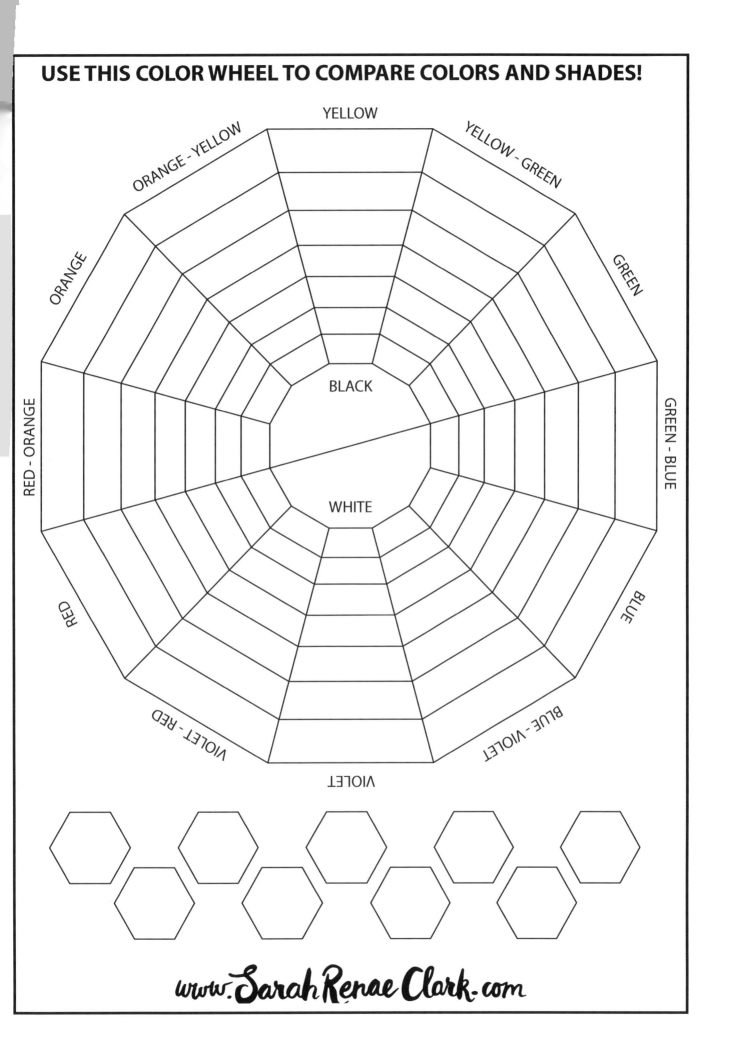

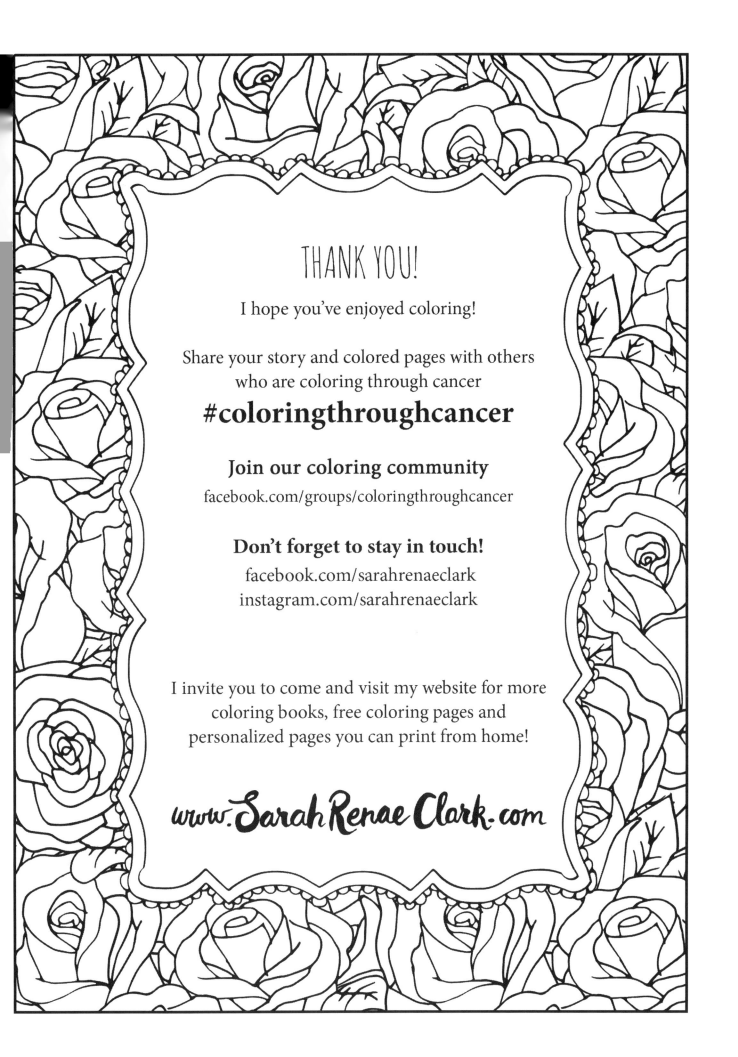

THANK YOU!

I hope you've enjoyed coloring!

Share your story and colored pages with others
who are coloring through cancer
#coloringthroughcancer

Join our coloring community
facebook.com/groups/coloringthroughcancer

Don't forget to stay in touch!
facebook.com/sarahrenaeclark
instagram.com/sarahrenaeclark

I invite you to come and visit my website for more
coloring books, free coloring pages and
personalized pages you can print from home!

www.SarahRenaeClark.com

Made in the USA
Las Vegas, NV
30 December 2022

64474536R10039